THE
ANTI-ANXIETY
TOOLKIT
Rapid Techniques to
Rewire the Brain

Melissa Tiers

ISBN: 978-1-466451-72-8
Bio photo: Julia Newman
Design: *www.trancepoetics.com*

To all my anxious clients,
students, and friends who trusted
me enough to let me into their
minds. Thank you.

TABLE OF CONTENTS

My goal for this little book is to allow the reader to be able to get relief within ten minutes of opening it. With that in mind, I'll keep this introduction short.

When I work with my clients to overcome anxiety, my approach is two-fold. First I teach them different techniques to address the cognitive, emotional/biochemical, structural and energetic aspects involved. For many people, just learning about these things decreases the intensity of episodes.

Then we work together to systematically neutralize the triggers

and reprogram the responses. So even though they have many techniques to stop anxiety, the reprogramming process makes it so
they rarely have to use them.

It's like learning a martial art. First, you learn how to kick ass. Then you learn how to never need to use it. It's interesting how the more skilled you get, the less you have to fight.

So, think of this book like that.

STOP THE BULLY
IN YOUR BRAIN

This book's preliminary chapters cover quick ways to interrupt the anxiety pattern. Once you get this you will be in a much more receptive state of mind to practice the more in depth processes that come later on.

Think of anxiety as a network of neural clusters in the brain that create an area of association — as some neuroscientists like to say, "the cells that fire together, wire together." For instance, a violin player will have an area of association that correlates to the hand she uses to finger the instrument. The more she practices, the more robust the area becomes. If she stops playing for a while, the cluster shrinks back to normal size. This corresponds to research on London taxi drivers that shows more density in the area of the brain associated with navigation. (Because unlike New York, London cabbies actually have to know the city.)

As you can see, the more we reinforce the pattern the thicker and stronger the cluster of neurons becomes. And as that happens, it becomes much more difficult to control them. My friend John Overdurf refers to these clusters of neurons as "the bully on the block who is strong, thick and overly sensitive. This makes it easily triggered."

But new research in neuroscience tells us that the brain is malleable and capable of changing even the most ingrained patterns. So, each time you stop the pattern of anxiety, you are working to rewire the brain. Google *neuroplasticity* if you want to learn more.

Luckily the brain can be rewired more easily than most people imagine, and by practicing all the techniques in this book you will become an expert in neuro-plasticity.

That's because if you can interrupt the anxiety and then connect that cluster to a more resourceful state like relaxation, you will be cross connecting those neurons and loosening up the area of association that had been keeping that cluster strong.

So not only do you get immediate relief, you are slowly but surely dismantling the neural network that used to keep that anxiety active.

And this book will give you many different ways to calm, inform, and change the bully in your brain.

Here's another way to think about it. Anxiety has a structure. Some people will see something external and then say something inside their heads and then feel anxious. Others will hear something or tell themselves something and then make an internal image and then feel anxious.

Other people will remember something as an image and then react to it by feeling anxious. There are many different combinations of the above.

Once you understand that you are generating the anxiety and that it doesn't just descend out of nowhere, you can begin to change it. This book will show you how to do that by changing the internal images, dialogue and feelings associated with it in the body.

We will start with quick and easy techniques to interrupt those patterns; we will then move towards all the different ways you can manipulate and change your internal strategies.

I suggest playing with and practicing these techniques as you read them. If you become familiar with them before the anxiety is in full swing, then you will be armed and ready when you need to be.

Bi-Lateral Stimulation

This technique involves stimulating both sides of the brain to stop anxiety. It is absurdly simple yet amazingly effective. Grab a ball (or apple or anything you can toss) and think of something that is causing you some anxiety.

When you can feel that anxiety somewhere in your body, rate the level of it on a scale of one to ten.

Now pass the ball back and forth, from one hand to the other, crossing the mid line, so you are stimulating both hemispheres of the brain. It will have a more rapid effect if you keep one hand in front of you as the other swings out to the side each time you pass the ball,. Do this for a minute. Stop. Take a deep breath, and check in. You might note that the anxiety has dissipated.

This is because by activating both hemispheres, you are spreading blood and electrical impulses throughout the brain and this floods that area of association and diffuses it. That bully of an anxiety cluster just can't keep itself together.

Now, think of the same situation again and see how much anxiety you can manage to conjure up, and rate it once again on the ten- to-one scale. Pass the ball or other object for a minute, and check in. Repeat till the anxiety has completely diffused.

This is something you can do anywhere. As soon as you start to feel that anxiety, simply grab an object — keys, a bottle of water, anything will work as long as you are moving both your arms, and crossing the mid-line of your body.

Peripheral Vision
(stop the world)

In helping people to overcome anxiety, I've noticed some commonalities. Whether it's what doctors call a specific or a generalized anxiety, internal dialogue is either the trigger or what keeps the pattern going.

You will learn many different ways to neutralize anxious internal dialogue later in this book, but for now, try this simple way of shifting out of your mind.

Start by picking a spot or focal point to stare at. Slowly begin to expand your peripheral vision to include all the space around the spot.

Now expand your vision even further to the sides, all the way up to the ceiling and down to the floor. Expand it even more, allowing your visual field to open so that you can imagine almost becoming aware of the space behind you.

This might feel strange at first but after practicing three or four times you will notice a general calm come over your mind and body as you realize your internal dialogue has stopped.

This is what Carlos Castaneda called "stopping the world." I teach it to my clients who have anxiety because it allows them to move awareness from the inside, out.

The great thing about peripheral vision is that it can be done anywhere, anytime and with practice, becomes another way of being in the world.

HEART COHERENCE

This technique is adapted from the work of the HeartMath Institute, which is a group of doctors and psychologists who are studying heart rate coherence and its effect on mental and physical health.

Start by bringing your awareness to your heart and as you do, imagine breathing deeply, in and out, from your heart. You might want to hold your hand over your heart to keep your awareness there as you breathe through it.

Imagine that as your heart is pumping healthy blood throughout your body, it is also radiating energy through your whole system.

The heart is the strongest emitter of electromagnetic energy in the body. By doing the exercise you are beginning to entrain your brain into a coherent and more relaxed brain-wave state.

The heart sends information to the brain in many ways: electromagnetically, which is how EKGs work; through the pulse, which sends information through a blood pressure wave; and biochemicaly, through releasing *atrial peptide*, a hormone that inhibits other stress hormones.

You can find out more by going to the *heartmathinstitute.com*.

Practice heart breathing throughout the day, knowing that as soon as you feel that anxiety you can drop immediately to your heart and breathe.

Sometimes, as you focus on your heart, you might want to think of someone or something that you love and allow that feeling to flow through your breathing.

And as you're feeling better, another thing that you might find interesting is to ask yourself, "What can I learn from this?"

You might be surprised by your answers.

A Jaw Dropping Moment

Another quick way to begin to take some of the power away from anxiety is to create a jaw dropping experience. Take a moment to relax your jaw as much as you can. Loosen it even more, and imagine it dropping to the floor.

Doing this stimulates the Vagus nerve which carries information from the nervous system to the brain, keeping it informed about what the body is doing. When you drop your jaw you are stimulating the parasympathetic nervous system to counteract the fight or flight response. And you are also encouraging the lungs to reach for a nice deep breath, creating a flood of the bio-chemicals associated with the relaxation response.

So relax your jaw, take a deep breath in, and pause for three counts. Then exhale twice as long through the nose. When you inhale deeply, put your hand on your belly and feel it rise. This ensures that you're breathing from your diaphragm.

Some people find that by inhaling to a count of four, pausing for three and exhaling for eight, they are able to keep their mind from ruminating as they allow the relaxation response to cohere with their breathing.

I find that after only three or four of these breaths, my clients are better able to do some of the slightly more involved techniques covered later in this book.

THE BACKWARD SPIN

One of the consistent things about anxiety and fear is that it's a physical feeling in the body. It's always moving, and usually it's moving too fast.

Think of the last time you got startled. You might remember the feeling starting somewhere in your body (for example, in your belly). It moves up (or down) and finally out as the fear passes through you.

But with anxiety, the fear moves up or down, but it doesn't move out. It keeps circulating through the body. This is why we say that fear has a spin.

This technique is a way to interrupt that cycle. It comes from Richard Bandler, the co-creator of Neuro-Linguistic- Programming (NLP) and can be used for many different uncomfortable emotional states.

Often I go through the exercise with my clients only once, and they are then able to use it on their own as a rapid way out of anxiety and into a far more resourceful state.

Here's how it works: locate where you feel the anxiety moving in your body, and notice which way the feeling spins. (It is often helpful to use your hand to model the direction of the spin.)

Next imagine that you can move the spin outside of your body. In other words, it's still spinning in the same way that you were feeling it before, but now it's outside of you.

Once you can feel it outside of yourself, reverse the spin (and the movement of your hand if you're using it).

As you do this, imagine bringing the spin back inside your body, rotating in this opposite direction. Notice how it feels different. Now, think of something funny and add some laughter to the spin because this will start to change the chemicals and hormones coursing through your body.

The next time you start to feel anxious, all you will have to do is notice the way it's spinning and reverse it. My clients report an immediate shift and some even feel a chuckle start to surface.

New Pathways

That freeze, fight or flight response
you go into during panic is mediated
by the unconscious mind. Your
breathing, heart rate and every other
system of your body is controlled
unconsciously. And lucky for us, it is.
Can you imagine having to remember
to breathe?

All of your habituated patterns,
emotional responses, long term
memory, cognitive filters and core
beliefs are in the domain of the
unconscious mind. This is why, when
you learn to use it strategically, you
will be able to change much faster.

Unconscious patterns and programs
are formed by repetition. Anything

done, felt or even imagined repeatedly begins to create habituated programs. Think about when you first learned to drive. It took all your conscious awareness to focus on steering and being aware of the gas, breaks, rearview mirror, speedometer and everything else you needed to pay conscious attention to. Then you drove for a while and before you knew it, your unconscious took over, and you found yourself chatting, daydreaming, eating, and listening to the radio—all while driving the car.

It's the same reason why they say you never forget how to ride a bike. It takes all your cognitive awareness to program the balance and fine motor skills involved in riding a bike, and once it's done, you never have to

consciously think about it again
because your unconscious rides the
bike. And although that's great for an
afternoon bike ride, it's not so great
when it triggers anxiety.

So think of these habituated patterns
like pathways in a forest. Every time
you feel anxious in certain situations
you are treading down a certain path.
One that is a little too easy for your
mind to traverse.

But as soon as you start using these
tools and feeling differently in those
same situations, it's like you are
cutting a new path.

At first it might be a bit difficult
because, just like in a forest, when

you cut a new trail, you have some clearing to do.

But every time you travel down this new path, every time you interrupt your old anxiety pattern, you are widening out that trail and it will get easier and easier for the mind to choose the new path as the old one begins to get overgrown.

Become the director
(Take One)

If you find yourself in a situation that provokes anxiety, imagine you could press the pause button, like when you watch a movie, and step out of it.

Once you step out, ask yourself how you would prefer to feel in this situation. Imagine trying on that better emotional state (like slipping on a coat of confidence or calm) and stepping back into the movie and noticing how it feels.

If it's still got some anxiety in it, step out again, and add more good feelings before stepping back in and trying it again.

Another way to do this is to imagine sending resources to yourself. Imagine the emotions you would rather have and then imagine you could transmit them to yourself in that movie.

If you can't access the emotion you want, sometimes it's easier to remember a time you felt that feeling and imagine seeing what you saw when you were there, hearing what you heard, and noticing how the feeling gets stronger inside you.

For example, if you want calm you can imagine it as a color and send it to yourself in that movie. Notice how the image of you takes in that calm and begins to relax in that movie scene. Imagine seeing your shoulders relax, your breathing shift, and your face reflecting an inner sense of calm.

If you want confidence, notice how your posture and expression shifts as you send yourself that confidence.

In your movie, once you feel the way you want to feel and look the way you want to look, imagine floating in and trying it on. Feel how good it feels to be in a body that feels good, even in that same situation that used to cause anxiety. Let your mind rehearse this new response, and with repetition you will rewire your brain.

BECOME THE DIRECTOR (TAKE TWO)

If it's a memory that's causing feelings of anxiety, notice what happens when you start to visualize the memory as if it were a movie. Notice what happens when you rewind it, speed it up, or slow it down; notice how you can turn it into an old, grainy, black and white movie to remind yourself that it's old and over.

Sometimes adding a silly sound track, like circus music, changes the way you respond to that memory. Sometimes this is all you need to neutralize the effect it was having on you.

You could, for example, make the movie smaller by shrinking it down or pushing it further away into the distance. You could change the characters in whatever way occurs to you. Make them silly or imagine them as little toddlers having tantrums.

One woman I worked with was having anxiety every time she had to speak with her boss. So, she decided to make a movie in which he was an angry and scared little boy whose parents never listened to him, throwing a tantrum to get attention. As you can imagine, visualizing him in this way changed the way she felt when she was around him.

If your family or co-workers are causing you anxiety, imagine a movie in which everyone is following a script—one that you wrote, edited, and are now directing.

For example, you could view a recent family interaction as if it were a scene from a Woody Allen movie. Or how about if David Sedaris wrote the script? Whatever comedic actor or writer you choose, notice how seeing that situation from their point of view allows you to shift perspectives—and hopefully see the irony in most family situations.

If that doesn't take the edge off, you can take this process a bit further by giving yourself more distance from the movie. This next idea comes from the work of Richard Bandler and John Grinder who developed what we call in NLP the *fast phobia cure*.

Here's how it works: imagine you are in the projection booth, watching yourself watching the movie, and from there manipulating it.

This makes the separation of emotion from the movie even more pronounced.

The first thing you want to do is to re-edit the movie by making sure the opening scene is neutral or safe.

For instance, if this were a memory or movie of a dog attack that led to a phobia, then the first scene would be

where you are safe, before
encountering the dog.

Then you want to edit in the last
scene where you are home, and it's
all over and you are safe. So the
movie goes from safe, to safe — with
the upsetting part in the middle.

So, from the projection booth, where
you're in total control of this movie,
see yourself in the theatre seat,
watching yourself in the movie.

And then watch the old grainy black
and white movie (with or without
silly soundtrack) and press pause
when you get to the end where
you're safe.

You can even rewind the movie
several times, watching everything
going in reverse and each time
imagining the quality of the film
degrading, getting older and grainier
with each viewing.

Some people imagine floating into the
movie when it's paused at the end,
and then experiencing everything
going in reverse.

You will notice how different it all
feels as you hear, feel, and see
everything going backwards.

You will know that you neutralized
the memory when you can watch it as
a movie, or think about the memory
and realize that your emotional
attachment to it has lost all its charge.

Shifting Perspective

You've learned how to locate the spin and reverse it. Now get ready to learn other fast ways to use metaphors and change the feeling.

As soon as you start to feel anxious, locate where it is in your body. As soon as you find it, notice the shape or other qualities of it and try playing with it. Change the shape and shrink it down and notice what happens.

Imagine it has a color. What color does it feel like? Now, what color would feel better? Imagine as you change the color to the one that feels better, that the anxiety changes into something else. What has it changed into?

Another way of feeling better is to imagine dropping right to the center of that anxiety and breathing through it. Notice what happens. As you drop to the center ask yourself, "If this were a message from my unconscious mind, what is it?" or "If there were a lesson here, what can I learn from this?"

You could imagine that anxiety as a pebble. Now imagine that pebble amongst many on a wide expansive beach. Now imagine that beach on an island. And that island in an ocean. On a planet….in a galaxy.

And notice how you feel now.

As you notice where in your body that anxiety is, you can ask yourself: "How do I want to feel instead?" Once you have an idea of an emotion you'd rather be feeling, talk yourself into it and notice how that better feeling moves in your body.

When you're feeling this better emotion, notice how differently you respond to any situation.

Here's what's going on under the hood: every emotional state has a set of biochemicals associated with it. When you have a certain biochemical state in the body, the brain generates more thoughts and emotions that are similar. It's as if you have a certain pair of colored glasses on so that everything you look at is colored by them.

When you are in a depressed state, everything seems depressing. Your past, present and future are all colored by that biochemical pair of shades you're wearing and it's really hard to see a better way or solution until you take the glasses off.

This is why most of these techniques involve a step off, or out, of the memory. This allows you to dissociate long enough for you to take those glasses off and think about a better biochemical state.

By asking yourself, "How do I want to feel instead?" you send the mind on a search for a better feeling state.

And once you find that better state, you have to get yourself to feel it. As you think yourself into that better emotional state, you can imagine that you are putting on a better or rosier pair of glasses through which to view your options or the situation. And notice how things change when the glasses come off, or change colors.

The Metaphoric Two-Step

Once you've located where in your body you feel the anxiety, ask yourself "what is this like?" and see what metaphor emerges.

One client of mine said her experience of anxiety was like a cauldron boiling over. I asked her what had to happen to change that and she said, "I have to turn off the flame and cool it down with ice."

I asked her to close her eyes and imagine doing that and notice what happens. She reported that the anxiety instantly cooled down.

Another client said her fear was like a big boulder stuck in her gut. I asked

her what has to happen in order for
that to change and she said, "I need
to break it up with
a drill."

Once she imagined doing that, she
said it turned to dust and
disappeared. As did her anxiety.

This sounds way too easy, I know. It
still surprises me that this process
works. But when you understand
that the unconscious mind speaks in
metaphor, you understand how
malleable our experience really is.

I challenge you to play with this.
When you start to feel anxious, notice
what its like and what metaphors or
symbols come to mind. Then imagine

a counter metaphor to change it, and
notice how much better you feel.

CHANGING INTERNAL DIALOGUE

The other way to change the pattern is to notice and manipulate the internal dialogue you are running that keeps that anxiety going.

As soon as you start feeling anxious, notice what you are saying to yourself. I guarantee it's not helpful and supportive. We are very good at feeding our anxiety by talking to ourselves in a really negative way. The good thing about realizing this is that you become more aware of all the things you would rather be hearing. And once you've become aware of this, you can begin to manipulate that negative self-talk.

Notice what happens when you hear
a negative statement in your mind
the way it normally is. Notice the
location of it. Is it coming from the
right, the left, in front of you, or
behind you? Switch it to the opposite
side and notice how it changes the
way you feel.

Now change the tempo, the tonality
or even the voice you hear it in. My
favorite is Minnie Mouse. When you
hear Minnie tell you, "you're not
good enough" or "you're just like
your father" in that high pitch squeal,
it just doesn't have the same effect.

Hear that negative self talk in the
voice of someone you would never
take seriously. Maybe some idiot

whose opinions you find laughable. For me it's a former president.

I had a client who was replaying a phrase told to her by her first boyfriend. And all these many years later, it was still making her feel worthless. So I asked her: now, as a grown woman, would you ever take to heart the words of a sixteen year old boy? As she laughed, the negative belief she had about herself seemed to evaporate.

Another client found that just by adding the word "so" to the beginning of her worry statements, the impact they had on her changed. She changed, "what if they don't like me?" to "so what if they don't like me?" And "what if I can't do this?" to "so what if I can't do this?"

Try this out. You might be surprised at how this simple two-letter word can change how you feel.

And try this: notice what happens when you take a negative statement and imagine it coming from the floor, the radio, or any other external place. Imagine a volume control and turn it down.

Nick Kemp, my friend and colleague, showed me a process where you find the negative statement associated to the anxiety and you repeat it in your head five times slower, separating the words from each other. And then repeat again, five times slower than that, and then again, five times slower, until the statement loses all of its negative charge.

You can also imagine reading that statement on a very large billboard, or on a sign being held by a cartoon character.

All these different ways of manipulating internal dialogue will help to make the statement absurd, unbelievable, or just plain boring. Once this happens, you'll realize that the anxiety doesn't have a way to keep going. You've interrupted the pattern and can now think about what you would rather hear yourself say inside your head.

Practice hearing that supportive voice or phrase. Try it from different angles and in different ways. Play with the tempo, tonality and volume and find what feels best to you.

DIAL IT DOWN

Now, having experimented with the tonality and volume control of your inner dialogue you might want to create a dial for anxiety that you can turn down when you need to.

When you start to feel anxious, immediately imagine a dial in your mind and notice what number it's turned to. Then imagine simply turning it down, and notice what happens.

In my office, I first always ask a client to turn the dial up a notch to allow the anxiety to increase a little bit. Once that happens, the mind has connected to the metaphor and it's easier to turn it down.

If I had asked my clients to just turn it down, they might not have believed it would work. I mean, if it was that simple, why the hell would they need me? They haven't realized that anxiety puts them into a highly suggestible state, and that's why the dial works. After all, they never have trouble turning it up.

To ensure that you are not turning up a powerful unpleasant state, make sure you try this when you are feeling only a mild state of anxiety. However once you get the dial set up, you can turn it down whenever you need to tune out that anxiety.

Relief is in your Hands

As anxiety comes on, many of my clients experience a tightening of muscles. As they become aware of this physical reaction, I ask them to notice the tension and imagine funneling it down into their hands as they make a tight fist.

I might say: Imagine every drop of that anxiety flowing into that fist and the more anxiety the tighter the fist. Once it has built up, and all the anxiety is contained in that hand, let it go. Imagine it flowing out or just dropping to the floor. You might even shake it out until that hand gets nice and loose.

If there is any left after you have let it go, simply send whatever is left down to that hand and repeat the process.

Sometimes the internal dialogue that's spinning in your mind can be transferred to that fist. As you let it go, imagine that dialogue loop *slooooowing* down and pouring right out of your hand along with that anxiousness.

Some people add a color to that tension and visualize it flowing down their arm, into their fist and then out their fingertips as they let it all go.

Some people hear the tension as it flows and peaks into the fist, and they imagine a whooshing sound as it leaves.

Go ahead and come up with your own variation that allows you to let it go even easier.

EMOTIONAL FREEDOM TECHNIQUE

This technique is one of my power tools. If there is one technique that you should spend some time experimenting with, this should be it.

Although extremely rapid in its ability to neutralize anxiety and the triggers that lead to them, it requires a bit more time to learn than the techniques in the previous chapter.

Emotional Freedom Technique, otherwise known as EFT, is a technique that involves tapping on powerful acupuncture points while redirecting the mind and conditioning in an anchor for a state of calm.

I was very skeptical of the claims that were being made about this technique, and so I spent years experimenting and challenging it. I will tell you that the first time I tried it I let go of a 30 year dental phobia. And the chronic migraine headaches I had most of my life are a thing of my past.

I never expect my clients to believe what I had a hard time believing myself, so I'll ask you to approach this with an experimenter's mind and try it on yourself. I'm giving you the short and fast version, referred to as Faster EFT because it seems to be more practical for my anxious clients. This variation was developed by Robert Smith and you can learn more from his free videos on his web site www.fastereft.com.

For a more in depth learning of this technique in its original form, go to www.emofree.com or (www.eftuniverse.com) where you can read the research as well as the hundreds of articles on different applications of EFT to a wide range of issues.

We start by setting an anchor for peace and calm. This is done by taking a moment to close your eyes and recreate a feeling of peace. Maybe you can imagine being on a beach or your favorite vacation spot, where you can remember, in as many senses as possible, hearing what you would hear, seeing what you would see and feeling how it feels to let go into relaxation. Maybe you can remember a yoga class

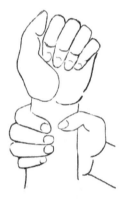

or meditation you once had and feel that calm. Whatever it takes to remind your body what peace and calm feel like.

When you access that internal state, take hold of your wrist with your hand so that your fingers are are wrapped around the inside and take a deep breath in and as you exhale slowly say to yourself "peace". Now you have an anchor. Some of my clients will use just this piece if they need it and are in an environment where tapping on their face wouldn't be appropriate. They simply grab their wrist, under their desk or wherever, take a deep breath in and slowly exhale as they think "peace" and they get a nice wave of calm.

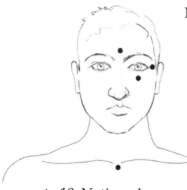

Now let's link it to the tapping of the acupuncture points. Start by tuning into the anxiety and assessing the intensity level on a scale of 0 to 10. Notice where you feel the anxiety in your body and then tap in between your eyebrows (your third eye) while saying "release and let go" Then tap on the side of the eye, under the eye and then your collar bone, all while repeating "I release and let this go". Then grab your wrist, take a deep breath in and as you slowly exhale say "peace". Now take a moment to reassess the intensity level. If there's still some anxiety, repeat the process as needed.

GOOD INTENTIONS

You already have so many amazing and rapid tools to stop anxiety and change the way you feel. Now we can explore a bit of what you can learn from having had that anxiety.

In NLP we have a saying that, "underneath every behavior is a positive intention." And I have found this idea to be extremely helpful in the way I approach change work.

Your unconscious mind is both adaptive and protective, and this means we have certain feelings for a reason. When we find out the reasoning we can work with it to find a better way to satisfy the underlying intention while letting go of the anxiety.

For example, imagine a child who, when asked to stand in front of his first grade class, didn't know the answer and so felt embarrassed and self-conscious.

The next time he is called to the front of the room, his brain immediately remembers the last time this happened, so he starts to get a little anxious. This causes him to go blank on the answer, and once again he feels embarrassed and his system is flooded with stress chemicals.

So of course he feels anxious if he even *thinks* of getting called on and he avoids raising his hand when he has a question for fear of feeling embarrassed. This reaction might cause him to have lower grades, thereby contributing to his anxiety and low self-esteem.

Now, as an adult, he has a phobia of public speaking. If he has to report in a board meeting, he begins to suffer anxiety. He might avoid any social situation where he might be the center of attention, and job interviews are a nightmare.

But his brain was only trying to protect him from feeling the initial stress and embarrassment. After all, it's a survival machine.

What happened is that when he went into the flight or flight response associated with anxiety, his brain took a virtual picture of the environment in order to prevent him from ever feeling it again. By creating anxiety the brain was hoping he would simply run away from the situation and be protected from the threat.

Unfortunately, running away from an angry boss or a question at a meeting isn't really an option. (However, the image of literally running away might be funny enough to spread some of the more happy hormones and biochemicals throughout the system.)

Still, it's useful to honor the subconscious in its attempt to protect us. And that's why many of the processes you're learning in this book involve asking the question, "what can I learn from this?" or "what's the message in this?"

Many times when my clients begin to act on the information they get from the answers to these questions, the anxiety dissipates.

For example, you can imagine having a dialogue with that anxiety and coming to some mutually beneficial way of changing the way you feel or act in certain situations.

Often manipulating all the pieces of the strategy gives you insights into the how and why of that anxiety.

Let's say you notice that every time you try to step into an elevator you have an instant image of your mother re-telling a horrible incident where she was trapped for hours in an elevator. You understand loud and clear why your unconscious is protecting you.

At this point you might try out one of the techniques you've already learned in this book. Once you're feeling better, you could create a movie of your mother and send her resources, or imagine swooping in and helping her escape from that situation.

Or maybe you'll want to do a round of EFT while stating, "even though I'm scared, I'm willing to let my mother's fear go."

Be creative. The possibilities are endless.

THE EMOTIVE JOURNEY

Another technique that can be informative and anxiety shifting, is called a "drop through" or "emotive journeying."

When you start feeling anxious, locate where it is in your body and imagine going right to the center of that feeling. Imagine it as a layer that you can drop through by asking yourself, "what's underneath this?"

Drop through and notice what feeling lies underneath; then drop through that by asking, "what's underneath this?" And keep going until you hit a good feeling or resource state. I know this sounds crazy, but all my clients

eventually uncover a powerful
positive state underneath it all.

Once you find the resource at the
core, underneath all the layers, then
allow yourself to soak it up. Imagine
it like an amazing, curative energy or
elixir and allow it to fill you up.

Once you are full of that core
essential state, imagine traveling back
up the layers, bringing this amazing
energy and noticing how it
transforms any negative state.

As you imagine and feel all those
emotions changing, notice how much
more powerful you feel; notice how
different that initial anxiety feels
now.

I love this process because it's a way of facing the fear head-on and discovering that when you do, it turns into something else. It shows the mind that when you stop running from it and dive right in with curiosity, you find you are far more resourceful than you ever imagined.

Taking it all in

You've been learning all different ways
to approach anxiety. You know how to
interrupt the cycle in the brain using bi-
lateral stimulation. You can tap it away
or change the feeling by spinning it
backwards. You can change the color,
shape or temperature; or you can just
breathe and drop through it.

You can change the internal dialogue by
slowing it down, changing volume,
tempo, tonality, and voice. You can slip
into peripheral vision and fade it out
completely and then begin to hear what
you would rather hear instead.

You can play with the memories by
making movies and messing around with
all the elements by pausing, rewinding,

adding soundtracks, editing, and
directing different outcomes.

You can learn from that anxiety by
dialoguing, dropping underneath it
or simply asking what the message is.

Take a moment and really think about
all of your resources and how many
different ways you can change.

Turn it around

The next method you will learn involves backing up the strategy to the beginning thought or belief that started it all.

One of my favorite cognitive approaches comes from the work of Byron Katie. It is simple, yet has profound effects. I strongly suggest taking some time to explore her work in depth by going to her web site *www.thework.com*

Basically, she believes that the only reason we suffer is because we *believe* the thoughts we are thinking. I completely agree and once you start to examine and challenge those thoughts as they are occurring, you will too.

If we are always walking around with different assumptions about ourselves and the world, and these beliefs either support us or make us feel bad, shouldn't we make sure they are at least valid thoughts?

Byron Katie does this by asking four questions and then doing what she calls a turn-around, which is a way of inverting the belief.

I have shortened the process to be even more effective in dealing with anxiety.

The first step is to determine the thought that is currently running through your head in the moment, or right before the anxiety. Simply ask yourself, "how am I thinking about this situation or myself that has me feeling anxious?"

For instance, one of my clients found that as she was about to go into a board meeting she was thinking, and believing the thought, "I'm a failure and can't do anything right." I asked her to notice how believing this thought made her feel and how that feeling made her act or react.

Next I had her ask herself, "can I absolutely know that this is true?" She had to really think about this.

Then I asked her to invert the thought. "I'm not a failure and I do many things right." And I asked her to come up with at least five examples of how this is true.

She said, "well, I got this job." And I said, good…that's one example where you didn't fail. (I also mentioned that she has a degree, so she didn't fail out of college.)

She then confessed that the last project she did for the company made a lot of money and got her a promotion. I said, that's three. Go on…

Well, she had raised two kids who were basically happy and successful. "And I've been supporting myself and my family for thirty years…"

We spent some more time going over all the different areas in her life, where she hadn't failed until she realized that the *opposite* of the belief that was causing her anxiety was so much truer for her. When this happens, the original negative belief loses most of its anxiety producing power.

It seems too simple and obvious, I know. But when you actually use it to counter one of your self-defeating beliefs, you'll realize it has a direct effect in how you feel.

Of course, sometimes you will find that the thought or belief really is true. In this case, confront your interpretation or reaction to this truth. As Byron Katie says, you are at

war with reality anytime you are
arguing with the things you or
someone else *should or shouldn't* be
doing. And is that really working for
you?

I have found that even for little
things, when I turn my thoughts
around it makes a big difference.
When I challenge the beliefs that
upset me or make me feel anxious,
my mind knows the routine and all I
have to do is ask myself, "is this
true?" And my emotions change.

SELF-HYPNOSIS TO REWIRE THE BRAIN

Being a clinical hypnosis instructor gives me a slightly different filter through which I study anxiety and all its varied responses. First and foremost, I see anxiety as a powerful state of hypnosis.

Because hypnosis conjures up many different ideas and misinformation abounds, I'll do my best to simplify and normalize the state so you'll understand how you slip in and out of it all the time.

You can think of hypnosis as a state of hyper-focused awareness, where the barrier that separates the conscious and the unconscious mind is pushed aside. This leads you into a state of heightened suggestibility.

For example, every time you get wrapped up in a good movie you slip into a state of heightened suggestibility. And without even trying, or being aware of it, you push aside that critical factor of the mind. It happens naturally. In movie language that is called *suspending disbelief*.

If you don't suspend disbelief when you sit down to enjoy a movie, you wouldn't be able to forget that you're watching a movie: there's an actor, there's a director, there's a producer and a whole sound crew; a camera crew, lighting crew, and all that stuff going on behind that camera. But we don't think about that. Unless of course, the movie stinks.

When you have a focused state of awareness combined with suspending disbelief, you will have that heightened state of suggestibility, where your unconscious mind is more receptive. And this is hypnosis.

This means that you jump when they want you to jump; you cry when they want you to cry.

Why? After all, you're intelligent. You know it's not real. There's somebody who wrote it. Somebody directed it. Somebody re-wrote it; somebody argued about the rewrites. It doesn't matter. For those two hours you are entranced.

An interesting feature of hypnosis is that on some level the brain doesn't know the difference between a real and an imagined event. So when the movie gets scary, your brain doses you with adrenaline, cortisol, and all the other stress hormones. Your heart beats faster and your breathing shifts. More blood goes to your arms and legs so that if you have to, you can fight or flight.

Unfortunately, the brain responds in the same way to our own internal movies — the ones that are made when you are imagining or worrying about doing something that makes you anxious.

That fear focuses awareness and in doing so pushes aside the rational critiquing part of the mind.

But when you imagine what it will feel like to feel better, your brain is rehearsing this state of mind. And this makes it so much easier to change that anxiety response if it happens to creep up in the future.

You can learn to go into a light hypnosis state and create new responses to those situations that used to cause anxiety.

Go ahead and start by getting comfortable and finding a spot to focus on. Then diffuse your focus and relax your vision

Then close your eyes and think "ten" as you imagine a wave of relaxation moving from the top of your head to the tips of your toes. Let it settle in with your breathing.

You will then open your eyes and close them as you think "nine," and add another wave of relaxation down your body. Some people imagine seeing the numbers fading and relaxing right out of their mind.

Open and close, "eight" and feel another layer of relaxation deepening this state of comfort. Allow every muscle to get even more relaxed as you continue counting down to one, opening and closing your eyes in between each count.

Then you can imagine a movie screen in your mind. This is your template upon which you can add or delete different scenes depending on what you would like to work on. You can make a movie where you see yourself being or reacting exactly the way you want to.

When it looks really good and compelling, you can float into that movie and into the you that has already started to change. Feel how good it feels to be doing what you want to be doing and feeling how you want to be feeling.

Then float back into your body, shake it off, and smile. You might do this quick and easy exercise daily, changing the movies to reflect all the different ways you want to change.

If you find that visualizing a movie and floating into it isn't easy for you, then you can simply imagine, after counting down, how you would feel if you had changed. Feel what it would feel like if you were free of that anxiety.

You might have an easier time talking to yourself in this relaxed state. You can say something like, "I feel relaxed and confident whenever I ..." And fill in where or when you want to be more comfortable.

If you are going to talk to yourself in this way, make sure you remember that the unconscious mind does not process negation very well. If I say "don't think of a blue elephant" what do you think of?

This means that if you say to yourself, "I don't want to feel anxious" or "I'm not going to panic" then the primary message to the unconscious mind is: "feel anxious" or "panic." So choose your message wisely. Make sure it's positive and in the present tense.

By practicing self hypnosis daily you will be conditioning in new responses to those triggers that used to cause anxiety. Think of it like programming your own internal GPS with a different set of directions.

◆◆◆

There are so many ways to step out of anxiety and into a better emotional state. I recommend you try them all out and feel which one makes sense for you.

So many people keep focusing on where they are instead of where they want to be. That's like programming your current location into the GPS and expecting to go somewhere. It doesn't work.

Luckily you've now got many tools in your kit designed to make the ride smoother. You're the one driving. Decide where you want to go and imagine how you want to feel — and soon you'll realize how much easier it is to keep your mind on the road in front of you.

ACKNOWLEDGEMENTS

This book is a collection of ideas I have been gathering from many brilliant minds over the years. I couldn't possibly list all the pioneers in neuroscience and mindbody medicine that have informed these pages, and so will simply thank all the researchers in neuroplasticity. Your work didn't just have an effect on the field, it changed the whole game.

I thank my favorite teacher, John Overdurf, who can be heard and felt throughout this book. A few daze with you and I had to re-write quite a few pages.....

Thanks to Richard Bandler and John Grinder who continue to find their way into everything I do.

Also thank you Jeffrey Schwartz, whose book *The Mind and the Brain* continues to have an amazing impact on my thoughts about change.

And finally thanks to Kristin Prevallet, writer and hypnotherapist, for taking this project away from me before I could overcomplicate it.

"

MELISSA TIERS is the author of the award winning
book "*Integrative Hypnosis: A Comprehensive Course in
Change.*" Founder of The Center for Integrative
Hypnosis, she maintains a private practice in New
York City while teaching classes in Integrative
Hypnosis, In-Depth NLP, Energy Psychology and
Mental Health Coaching. Melissa has advanced
certifications in both clinical hypnosis and alternative
healing; she is an adjunct faculty member of The Open
Center and the Tri-State College of Acupuncture.

If you would like to learn more about Melissa's training
schedule or would like to sponsor a workshop, go to
www.melissatiers.com.
For a full online video course of this protocol, go to:
www.centerforintegrativehypnosis.com

PRAISE FOR *Integrative Hypnosis:*
A Comprehensive Course in Change
BY MELISSA TIERS

I cannot stress enough what a valuable resource
this book is! It doesn't matter whether you are a
psychiatrist, therapist, just curious about hypnosis,
or are looking for relief from your own symptoms
— this book will prove to be a wonderful and
powerful tool for you.

Melissa manages to transport the reader into
her "virtual" classroom where Milton Erickson,
Bandler & Grinder and so many more of the great
healers of our time will share their unique healing
genius through her wonderful teaching style. She
also gives the reader full access to her own unique
knowledge and use of these powerful healing arts;
access that would normally cost a person
thousands of dollars in workshop/seminar fees.

Melissa makes powerful healing techniques seem so easy to learn and incorporate into your practice (if you're a professional healer as I am) and by keeping it simple, allows anyone with an interest to understand how to help themselves and others. Navigating the "mind field" never felt so natural or easy until I read this book. Thank you Melissa for yet another wonderful gift!

- JACK CLEARY MS, MEd
  CLINICAL THERAPIST & CERTIFIED HYPNOTIST

◆◆◆

As a Columbia-trained psychiatrist, I thought I knew a thing or two about therapy. Five years ago, I had my first training in hypnosis with Melissa Tiers, and she immediately began to blow my mind with her challenging perspectives, attuned teaching, and powerful hypnotic skills. Her influence has transformed the way I practice psychiatry, and many of my patients have been the direct benefactors. Hypnosis, NLP, and EFT have become some of the most powerful modalities in my clinical toolbox, and very few clinicians come close to Melissa's versatility in utilizing and teaching these skills. Her book is a faithful, you-are-there rendering of her trainings, complete with the charm, wit, and playfulness that Melissa infuses into her work. She remains one of the most talented, creative, and generous human beings I've ever encountered, and this book is a gift that I'm sure you and your clients will benefit from. And now, you can take a deep breath, relax into a smile, notice how the pages turn effortlessly, as you absorb the wisdom of an expert teacher...

- ANTHONY J. TRANGUCH MD PHD
  PRIVATE PRACTICE PSYCHIATRIST & ASSISTANT
  CLINICAL PROFESSOR OF PSYCHIATRY, COLUMBIA
  UNIVERSITY

♦♦♦

There are books that should be required reading for anyone with an interest in healing with hypnosis and *Integrative Hypnosis: A Comprehensive Course in Change* by Melissa Tiers is one of them. What makes her truly comprehensive training so special is the ease and grace in which Melissa empowers you to apply what you learn as soon as you finish each chapter. When you finish this fun-filled learning experience you will have a functional toolbox for assisting clients with confidence.

I think this book is outstanding—Great job Melissa!

-MICHAEL ELLNER MSH, CHT
MEDICAL HYPNOTIST AND HYPNOSIS EDUCATOR
BEDSIDE MANNERS: THE PAIN CLINICIAN'S GUIDE TO EFFECTIVE MEDICAL COMMUNICATION

◆◆◆

Integrative Hypnosis: A Comprehensive Course in Change is without equal — period....The greatest bonus here is that while you could go out and buy fifty or a hundred books on hypnosis, NLP and other approaches, then spend years reading and wading through them, you could just buy this book now and have Melissa blend all that knowledge into a process that is at once enlightening and refreshing.

Whether you are just curious about hypnosis or already a professional practitioner; get this book. It is awesome! Just like the author.

-DAN CLEARY, HYPNOSIS INSTRUCTOR, PAIN RELIEF EDUCATOR; AUTHOR OF *TARGETING PAIN: A PRACTITIONERS GUIDE TO RELIEF*

◆◆◆

Melissa Tier's book is not only educational, it is an eye-opening read that intrigues the reader to

practice the methods taught. As a student of Melissa's in her certified integrative hypnosis course, I was able to get support and information from the book which reads like one of her classes. Her book outlines in detail how to effectively practice hypnotherapy. She is an excellent and dynamic teacher who loves teaching integrative hypnosis as well as EFT and NLP modules. Great read! She is a wonderful healer and enthusiastic professor of hypnosis!
- JENNIFER HAUS, LCSW, CH

This book is a wonderful cornucopia of current and relevant information in the field of hypnosis and beyond — as synthesized by an outstanding hypnotist and brilliant thinker and innovator in the field of hypnosis, Melissa Tiers. I am a licensed clinical social worker with more years in the field than I wish to disclose! After an extended period of fatigue in my work, I had the opportunity to study with Melissa, and she has given me the inspiration to continue my work — in new and exciting ways. Melissa is truly a walking encyclopedia of information, which is well reflected in this book, and I believe it serves as a great resource for any professional wanting to invigorate their practice with creative, practical and very user friendly tools. There are some chapters of my personal copy of the book which I have literally discolored from all the yellow pen highlighting!

The book reads in the manner in which Melissa teaches — a meandering journey, which in itself, is evocative of both the classroom experience, as well as a subtle (or not so subtle) elicitation of the more unconscious, creative processes. And yet, she also manages to make what might seem quite amorphous (the creative, unconscious mind, for example) feel like the most pragmatic and obvious tool for self

healing. (And with all that we are learning these days from the world of neuroscience, I believe, indeed, that these are some of the most potent strategies currently available to us!) That's a big part of what makes her so talented — her ability to make the complex quite accessible and usable. My only criticism is that Melissa is quite dynamic in person, and she has a great instructional DVD, which I also use as a reference tool. Perhaps in her next edition of the book she will add an audio and/or DVD component as well.... that's just a suggestion!
- MARTHA E. MILLER, LCSW

♦♦♦

The book is written in the style in which Melissa teaches – clear, succinct, pragmatic, and rich with vignettes that make the material accessible to both the novice and seasoned practitioner. I speak from first-hand experience as one who was a traditionally trained psychiatrist who felt that long term therapy and/or psychotropic medications alone were limited options in addressing the problem of people who came to see me. I felt a need to add to my existing skill set by seeking further training in hypnosis, stress management, pain control, the management of post-traumatic stress disorder, creative usage of language, and other tools that could be incorporated into clinical practice. Enter, Melissa Tiers.

Having had the privilege of being trained by Melissa I can say with assurance that she possesses a rare ability to effortlessly transform theory into practice. Her knowledge base in the field is encyclopedic; her enthusiasm contagious; her ability to clarify complex concepts in a simple and therapeutically relevant manner is exemplary. Couple that with an incisive sense of humor that gets appropriately integrated into her interventions, and a sensitivity to recognize and resonate with the best learning styles for each of her students. You are in for a life-enriching experience.

- HENRY SPITZ M.D.; D.F.A.P.A.
  CLINICAL PROFESSOR OF PSYCHIATRY
  COLUMBIA UNIVERSITY, COLLEGE OF PHYSICIANS & SURGEONS
  DISTINGUISHED LIFE FELLOW, AMERICAN PSYCHIATRIC ASSOCIATION